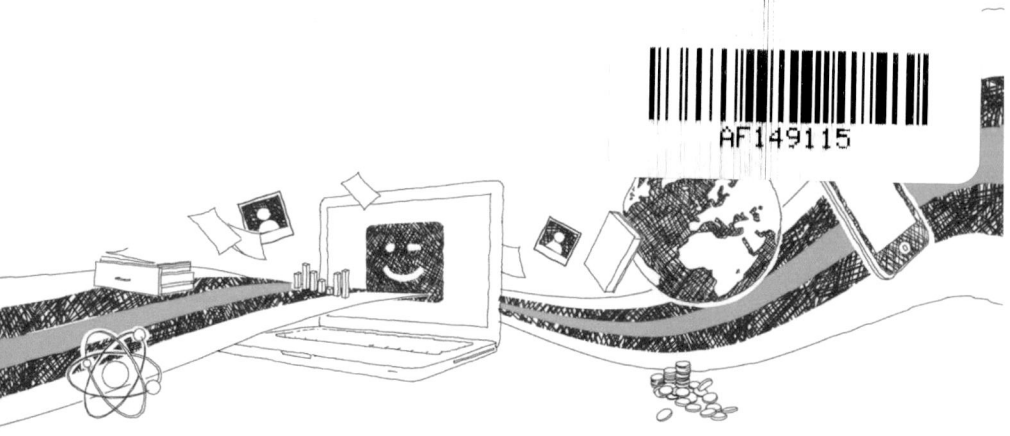
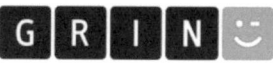

Patrick Kimuyu

Improving Hand Hygiene Compliance by Healthcare Workers

GRIN Publishing

GRIN - Your knowledge has value

Since its foundation in 1998, GRIN has specialized in publishing academic texts by students, college teachers and other academics as e-book and printed book. The website www.grin.com is an ideal platform for presenting term papers, final papers, scientific essays, dissertations and specialist books.

Visit us on the internet:

http://www.grin.com/

http://www.facebook.com/grincom

http://www.twitter.com/grin_com

IMPROVING HAND HYGIENE COMPLIANCE BY HEALTHCARE WORKERS

Name: Patrick K. Kimuyu
University: Egerton University

Hand hygiene has emerged as the only single strategy that has the potential for reducing hospital-acquired infections. Evidence indicates that hospital-acquired infections pose an immense hazard for patients within the hospital environment, and healthcare workers, including nurses are involved in the transmission of these infections (Pittet, Allegranzi & Boyce, 2009). According to World Health Organization [WHO] (2010), the prevalence and incidence of hospital-acquired infections among the global population has been increasing with more than 1.4 million people suffering from these infections, worldwide. Evidence indicates that transmission of hospital-acquired infections from patient to patient occurs often through the hands of healthcare workers (Al-Busaidi, 2013). This implies that enhancing hand hygiene among healthcare workers holds the potential for reducing and preventing hospital-acquired infections. In most cases, patients experience hospital-acquired infections during their hospital stay, but appearance after discharge has been reported. Additionally, hospital-acquired infections affect hospital staff as occupational infections. In Australia, hospital-acquired infections are considered as one of the issues that threaten patient safety. This phenomenon has been reported worldwide. As reported by Huis et al. (2012), 4.6 to 9.3% of hospitalized patients in Europe are affected by hospital-acquired infections, accounting for about 135,000 deaths, whereas 99,000 hospital-acquired infections-associated deaths occur in the US, annually. As such, hand hygiene is considered as a significant preventive approach for reducing hospital-acquired infections. This explains why health organizations such as WHO, The Joint Commission and Centers for Disease Control have embarked on spearheading education and awareness on hand hygiene (Pittet, Allegranzi & Boyce, 2009; The Joint Commission, 2009). Despite these efforts, evidence indicates that healthcare workers continue to exhibit low levels of hand hygiene compliance (Erasmus et al., 2010). Therefore, this essay will demonstrate how nurses can assume a leadership role within the hospital settings in accordance with the health safety standards (National Safety and Quality Health Services) as outlined by the Australian Commission on Safety and Quality in Health Care [ACSQHC]. I will discuss how nurses can adopt hand hygiene strategies to improve compliance to the national hand hygiene initiative in the wards as one of the key approaches for preventing and controlling hospital-acquired infections.

Despite extensive efforts to improve hand hygiene among healthcare workers, the rates of hand hygiene compliance have not been optimal. However, it is apparent that different groups of healthcare workers demonstrate varied hand hygiene compliance levels. In one cross-sectional study that was carried out by Chavali, Menon and Shukla (2014), nurses were found to have hand hygiene compliance rate compared to compliance rate of other

2

healthcare workers. Based on the WHO hand hygiene guidelines, overall compliance for participants in this study was high. This implies that compliance rates for nurses were relatively lower than the WHO guidelines. Additionally, nurses recorded the lowest hand hygiene compliance before aseptic procedures in the surgical Intensive Care Unit. Therefore, findings of this study explains the rationale for adopting appropriate hand hygiene strategies which can improve nurses' compliance to hand hygiene guidelines in the wards as one of the main approaches of improving patient safety. On the other hand, hand hygiene compliance enhances the implementation of the Australian national healthcare standards related to patient safety. The ACSQHC (2012) outlines the national safety and quality health service standards which are meant to improve patient safety. Specifically, *Standard 3*: focuses on reducing hospital-acquired infections across the continuum of healthcare. Therefore, nursing leadership approaches can have a significant contribution to health safety through hand hygiene given that nurses constitute the largest portion of the Australian healthcare workforce (Twigg, Duffield & Evans, 2013).

Multi-modal educational strategy is the first hand hygiene strategy that can improve compliance among nurses, as well as other healthcare workers. Over the decades, education has been adopted as one of the main strategies for improving compliance to hand hygiene guidelines. Overall, knowledge is very essential in the healthcare profession. As such, adopting educational programs on hand hygiene can help in enhancing hand hygiene compliance among healthcare workers, including nurses. In practice, disease preventive and control interventions are designed and taught to healthcare workers through education and training. Therefore, theoretical knowledge on hand hygiene is essential for medical students, as well as professional healthcare workers. However, evidence indicates that knowledge about hand hygiene among medical students is not adequate. According to Prabhakumar et al. (2016), medical students exhibit sub-optimal knowledge on hand hygiene. In this study, knowledge levels on hand hygiene among medical students were found to be far below the expected levels based on the WHO guidelines. As a result, they recommend the inclusion of hand hygiene in the educational curricula, an aspect that has not been implemented in Australia. Instead, nurses, as well as the other healthcare workers acquire much of the hand hygiene knowledge at their workplace during their professional practice. This explains the need for further education and training on hand hygiene within the clinical setting.

From a critical perspective, the effectiveness of multi-modal educational strategy in enhancing hand hygiene compliance among healthcare workers has been studied extensively. According to Martín-Madrazo et al. (2009), there is sufficient evidence that educational programs on hand hygiene are effective in improving compliance to national regulations and international protocols which are aimed at reducing hospital-acquired infections. These educational programs achieve their efficacy for improving hand hygiene compliance through increasing the knowledge regarding hand hygiene among healthcare workers. They also promote positive attitudes regarding hand hygiene among healthcare workers, an aspect that improves compliance to international protocols and national regulatory guidelines.

Evidence on the effectiveness of multi-modal educational programs regarding hand hygiene compliance can be provided by a cross-sectional study that was carried out in Bangladesh. In this study, Ara et al. (2014) investigated the effectiveness of this strategy in reducing hospital-acquired infections based on compliance to hand hygiene guidelines. The objective of this study was to improve hand hygiene compliance among healthcare workers as a reliable approach for controlling and preventing hospital-acquired infections. These investigators used an educational/training intervention to raise awareness on the significance of hand hygiene among healthcare workers, primarily nurses and physicians. The findings of this study indicated that education and training improves compliance to hand hygiene guidelines among healthcare workers. Overall compliance was found to increase compliance with nurses recording a higher compliance compared to physicians. Additionally, education serves as the most appropriate approach for passing emerging research knowledge to professional nurses, as well as other healthcare workers. Over the past decades, healthcare transformation has been based on evidence-based practice whereby new evidence from research is transformed into practice within the clinical setting (Stevens, 2013). In the same way, hand hygiene guidelines which have been developed through evidence-based approaches can be introduced into nursing practice through educating nurses on new knowledge regarding this preventive practice.

Teaching programs based on hand hygiene guidelines are being developed. For instance, WHO has developed a multi-modal educational program based on what is referred to as "My 5 Moments for Hand Hygiene". This approach focuses on improving patient safety by preventing and controlling hospital-acquired infections. It encourages hand hygiene during five critical moments; before touching a patient, after touching a patient and patient's surroundings, before aseptic procedures, and after exposure to body fluid (WHO, 2010). This educational program has been found to be effective in improving hand hygiene compliance among healthcare workers, including nurses. In the recent quasi-experimental trial that was carried out by Farhoudi et al. (2016) who investigated the impact of WHO's multi-modal hand hygiene strategy in 14 hospital wards. Investigators in this study carried out an educational intervention that involved hand hygiene teaching sessions based on the WHO's five moment program and assessed its impact on compliance over 12 months. Nurses were enrolled in hand hygiene related educational courses. According to the findings of this study, compliance among nurses increased significantly after intervention. Similarly, compliance among doctors increased following the intervention. This demonstrates that educational programs improve compliance to hand hygiene protocols among nurses.

The second strategy that can improve hand hygiene among nurses is the behavioral changes strategy as it is demonstrated by health workers' behavior for using of hand hygiene products. This strategy enhances the use of hand hygiene products among healthcare workers. Evidence indicates that hand hygiene products such as alcohol-based solutions, paper towels, antiseptic gels and soaps are commonly used in most hospitals and other healthcare facilities. Canham (2011) recommends the use alcohol-based hand-rub in clinical settings due to their effectiveness in decontaminating hands. The effectiveness of hand hygiene products has been investigated and confirmed to improve compliance among healthcare workers. In one prospective study that was carried out by Mu et al. (2016) that investigated the impact of hand hygiene intervention on compliance, the use of hand hygiene was found to improve compliance. Investigators in this study investigated the consumption of hand hygiene products per patient-day before and after intervention and compared it with the rates of hospital-acquired infections. Overall, findings of this study indicated that hand hygiene compliance among healthcare workers improved after intervention. Other studies have investigated the effectiveness of various hand hygiene products. These studies reveal that alcohol-based hand hygiene products demonstrate high efficacy for hand decontamination. For instance, Girou et al. (2002) tested the efficacy of alcohol-based solution versus antiseptic soap. Investigators in this study concluded that alcohol-based solutions are more efficient in hand decontamination than antiseptic soaps. The efficacy of these alcohol-based solutions is based on their ability to denature microbial proteins leading to the eradication resident and transient microflora. Ideally, alcohol-based hand hygiene solutions are supposed to have 60% to 95% alcohol concentration, in order to demonstrate high potency. Higher alcohol concentrations are considered to be less potent due to low water content which is essential for the denaturing of microbial proteins of the pathogens (Kampf & Loffler, 2010).

From a critical perspective, both multi-modal and behavior changes strategies improve compliance among healthcare workers in various ways. For instance, multi-modal educational strategy improves compliance through four main approaches. Foremost, it enables nurses and other healthcare workers to update their knowledge on hand hygiene.

Training nurses on new hand hygiene techniques increases their ability to adhere to hand hygiene guidelines. Second, multi-modal educational hand hygiene strategy plays a pivotal role in promoting positive attitudes towards hand hygiene among nurses. In theory, compliance to international and national regulations in healthcare is influenced by social behaviors. Positive attitudes are associated with increased compliance. In contrast, negative attitudes among healthcare workers are associated to poor compliance. The third way through which education improves compliance is through creating awareness on the importance of hand hygiene. Nurses, as well as other healthcare workers are taught about the emerging techniques that increase the control and prevention of hospital-acquired infections within the clinical setting. Finally, hand hygiene educational strategy plays a significant role in improving practice. In the context of nursing practice, this strategy informs nurses' decisions on patients' care, leading to improved patient outcomes. On the other hand, hand hygiene products increase compliance due to their ease of application compared to other hand hygiene strategies. The use of hand hygiene products is reported to be time-saving. They take little time to decontaminate hands. For instance, hand decontamination with alcohol-based hand-rubs takes between 15 to 30 seconds (Canham, 2011). As such, healthcare workers prefer this strategy because it requires less time, an aspect that improve compliance. Second, it is reported that alcohol-based hand-rubs are convenient for hand cleaning among healthcare workers. These alcohol-based solutions have been reported to reduce skin irritations (Kampf & Loffler, 2010); thus, increasing occupational safety of healthcare workers.

Overall, hand hygiene emerges as one of the main aspects related to patient safety which is reinforced by national standards. Infection Control Department has the responsibility of ensuring patient safety, especially through reducing the prevalence of hospital-acquired infections. In this context, education and the use of hand hygiene strategies are consistent with the national standards. According to ACSQHC (2012), healthcare facilities are expected to adopt effective strategies for preventing and controlling hospital-acquired infections. Specifically, *Standard 3.5* requires healthcare facilities to develop, implement and audit hand hygiene programs based on the national hand hygiene initiative. This involves regular auditing of hand hygiene compliance by the workforce, reporting of compliance rates to the highest level of organizational governance and adopting appropriate measures to address non-compliance to hand hygiene guidelines. In this case, educating and training nurses on hand hygiene, as well as encouraging the use of hand hygiene products such as alcohol-based solutions, antiseptic soaps, foams and gels are some of the most appropriate hand hygiene strategies that can increase compliance among nurses in the wards. This can lead to a significant decrease in the prevalence of hospital-acquired infections.

In retrospection, it is apparent that improving hand hygiene compliance has significant implications to nursing practice. Foremost, it prevents the occurrence of hospital-acquired infections; thus, improving patient safety, the core goal of nursing practice. Second, hand hygiene reduces the spread of antimicrobial resistance. Hand hygiene compliance has been found to reduce methicillin-resistant *S. aureus* (MRSA) and *Clostridium difficle* (Mathur, 2011). Antimicrobial resistance has emerged as the single most factors that hinder prevention and control of infections. Nursing practice seeks to adopt evidence-based nursing interventions to improve the patients' quality of life through the provision of effective nursing care. As such, any approach that is proven to achieve this objective such as hand hygiene is considered to advance the development of nursing practice. Finally, nursing care aims at reducing infections through safe practice and hand hygiene promotes safe nursing care. Therefore, hand hygiene serves as a reliable approach for reducing antimicrobial resistance.

Implementation of multi-modal educational and behavioral changes strategies can be achieved through various ways. The Infection Control Department can develop institutional guidelines that promote hand hygiene education and use of hand hygiene products among nurses. Maxfield and Dull (2011) consider this department as a partner, resource and enforcer. However, Cambell (2010) observes that responsibility of hand hygiene does not rest on the Infection Control Department, but also other stakeholders such as nursing leaders and hospital administration. On the one hand, up-to-date education sessions and training for nurses regarding hand hygiene can improve compliance (Hart, 2013). Additionally, promotional materials, especially posters explaining the importance of hand hygiene should be placed in noticeable areas in the wards (Smith & Lokhorst, 2009). On the other hand, increasing the availability of hand washing sinks and hand hygiene products in the wards can enhance the implementation of these strategies. However, implementing these hand hygiene products involves some barriers. Chagpar et al. (2010) identifies attitudinal and process barriers. Attitudinal barriers are related to nurses' unwillingness to comply with the proposed hand hygiene. On the other hand, process barriers involve institutional guidelines that interfere with hand cleaning. For instance, nurses are expected to wear gloves before touching patients, the same moment when decontamination should be done based on the WHO's five moments. Other barriers include lack of institutional commitment, availability of hand hygiene facilities and work overload among nurse (Martín-Madrazo et al., 2009).

In a brief conclusion, hand hygiene compliance is usually low among nurses. However, the use of hand hygiene interventions such as multi-modal and behavioral changes strategies improves compliance. They improve compliance through increasing nurses' knowledge regarding hand hygiene, building competence and promoting the development of positive attitudes. Therefore, these strategies can be implemented in wards to improve compliance to the NSQHS standards. However, implementation can be impaired by attitudinal and process barriers.

References

Al-Busaidi, S. (2013). Healthcare workers and hand hygiene practice: a literature review. *Diffusion: the UCLan Journal of Undergraduate Research, 6*(1), 1-13.

Ara, L., Mowla, S., Mahmud, S., & Mahmud, A. R. (2014). Effectiveness of education and training in improving hand hygiene compliance among the healthcare workers at a community based healthcare setting in Bangladesh. *The 9th Healthcare Infection Society Conference International Conference.* doi:10.13140/RG.2.1.3506.1363

Cambell, R. (2010). Hand-washing compliance goes from 33% to 95% steering team of key players drives process. *Healthcare Benchmarks and Quality Improvement, 17*(1), 5-6.

Canham, L. (2011). The first step in infection control is hand hygiene. *The Dental Assistant,* 42-46.

Chavali, S., Menon, V., & Shukla, U. (2014). Hand hygiene compliance among healthcare workers in an accredited tertiary care hospital. *Indian J Crit Care Med., 18*(10), 689–693.

Erasmus, V., Daha, T., & Brug, H. (2010). Systematic review of studies on compliance with hand hygiene guidelines in hospital care. *Infect Control Hosp Epidemiol., 31,* 283–94.

Farhoudi, F., Dashti, A., Davani, M., Ghalebi, N., Sajadi, G., & Taghizadeh, R. (2016). Impact of WHO Hand Hygiene Improvement Program Implementation: A Quasi-Experimental Trial. *BioMed Research International, 2016,* 7026169.

Girou, E., Loyeau, S., Legrand, P., Oppein, F., Brun-Buisson, C. (2002).Efficacy of hand rubbing with alcohol based solution versus standard hand washing with antiseptic soap: randomized clinical trial. *BMJ, 325*(7360), 362.

Hart, T. (2013). Promoting hand hygiene in clinical practice. *Nursing Times, 109,* 38, 14-15.

Huis, A., Achterberg, T., Bruin, M., Grol, R., Schoohoven, L., & Hulscher, M. (2012). h12A systematic review of hand hygiene improvement strategies: A behavioral approach. *Implementation Science, 7,* 92.

Kampf, G. & Loffler, H. (2010). Hand disinfection in hospitals-benefits and risks. *Journal of the German Society of Dermatology, 8*(12), 978-983.

Martín-Madrazo, C., Cañada-Dorado, A., Salinero- Fort, M., Abanades-Herranz, J., Arnal-Selfa, R., García-Ferradal, I.,… Soto-Diaz, S. (2009). Effectiveness of a training program to improve hand hygiene compliance in primary healthcare. *BMC Public Health, 9,*469.

Mathur, P. (2011). Hand hygiene: Back to the basics of infection control. *Indian J Med Res., 134*(5), 611–620.

Maxfield, D. & Dull, D. (2011). Influencing hand hygiene at spectrum health. *Physician Executive Journal, 37*(3), 30-34.

Mu, X., Xu, Y., Yang, T., Zhang, J., Wang, C., Liu, W.,...Chen, J. (2016).Improving hand hygiene compliance among healthcare workers: an intervention study in a Hospital in Guizhou Province, China. *Braz J Infect Dis., 20*, 5.

Pittet, D., Allegranzi, B., & Boyce, J. (2009). The World Health Organization Guidelines on Hand Hygiene in Health Care and their consensus recommendations. *Infect Control Hosp Epidemiol., 30*, 611–22.

Prabhakumar, D., Chakravarthy, M., Nayak, S., Hosur, R., Padgaonkar, S., Harivelam, C., & Bharadwaj, A. (2016). Knowledge levels of medical students about hand hygiene. *J Nat Accred Board Hosp Healthcare Providers, 3*, 27-31.

Smith, J.M. & Lokhorst, D.B. (2009). Infection control: can nurses improve hand hygiene practice? *Journal of Undergraduate Nursing Scholarship, 11*(1), 1-6.

The Australian Commission on Safety and Quality in Healthcare. (2012). *National safety and quality health service standards*. Sydney, Australia: ACSQHC.

The Joint Commission. (2009). *Measuring hand hygiene adherence: overcoming the challenges. 1st ed.* Oakbrook Terrace, IL: The Joint Commission.

Twigg, D., Duffield, C., & Evans, G. (2013). The critical role of nurses to the successful implementation of the National Safety and Quality Health Service Standards. *Australian Health Review, 37*, 541-546.

WHO (2010). *A guide to the Implementation of the WHO multimodal hand hygiene improvement strategy*. Geneva, Switzerland: WHO.

YOUR KNOWLEDGE HAS VALUE

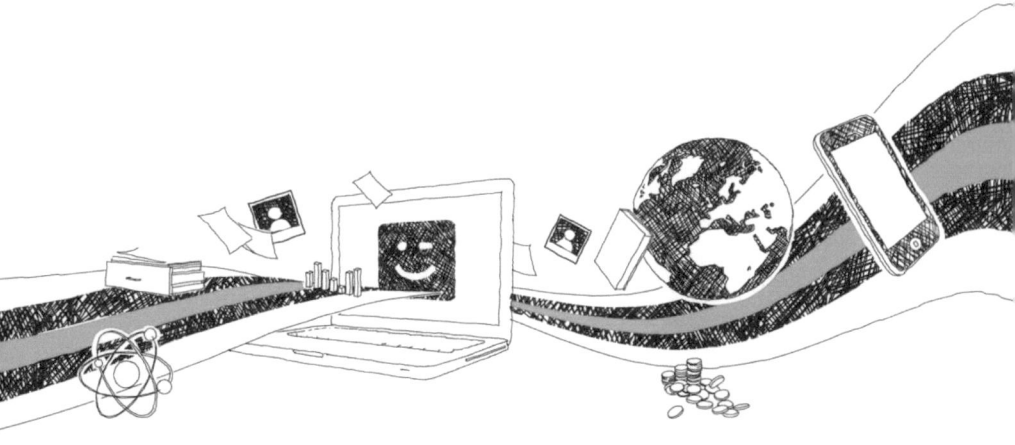

- We will publish your bachelor's and
  master's thesis, essays and papers

- Your own eBook and book -
  sold worldwide in all relevant shops

- Earn money with each sale

Upload your text at www.GRIN.com
and publish for free

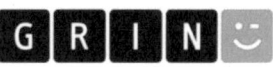

Bibliographic information published by the German National Library:

The German National Library lists this publication in the National Bibliography; detailed bibliographic data are available on the Internet at http://dnb.dnb.de .

Imprint:

Copyright © 2017 GRIN Verlag, Open Publishing GmbH
Print and binding: Books on Demand GmbH, Norderstedt Germany
ISBN: 9783668563766

This book at GRIN:

http://www.grin.com/en/e-book/378995/improving-hand-hygiene-compliance-by-healthcare-workers